MY CHILD HAS BEEN DIAGNOSED WITH ADHD

Attention Deficit Hyperactive Disorder

Ernest L. Sanders
A Clinical Mental Health Counselor

Acknowledgement

This book is dedicated to the greatest therapist on the planet earth located at

L. Williams and Associates
Birmingham, Alabama

Table of Content

My Child Has ADHD………………………………………….……..4

FEAR……………………………………………………………..…….8

ADHD……………………………………………………………...…..10

Psycho-therapy for parent and child……………………………..…12

Medication………….…………………………………………….…..15

Conclusion……………………………………………….…………..22

Resources……………………………………………………….…...23

My Child Has been diagnosed ADHD

Thank you for reading this book. The intention of the author is to give you a simple down to earth understanding of a complicated diagnosis-ADHD. As of the date of this writing there is no known cure for ADHD, but you can control ADHD. You will need the help of other professionals, a great deal of patience and the receiving of correct information. In many instances, child outgrow ADHD. It is important that each parent seek correct information concerning ADHD, its cause, symptoms, diagnosis and treatment. Yes, your neighbor has good information; your mom has good information, in fact all the information you can gather whether on the internet or from family friends and neighbors is important and useful. Bad information helps you find good information and good information helps your better help your child. No information is bad but every situation is different. You need information designed for your special child. Get a professional to help put together your tailored made plan for your special situation.

Those acronyms ADHD stand for Attention-Deficit Hyperactive-Disorder. ADHD is a mental disorder diagnosed by a professional after review and clinical evaluation. ADHD (attention-deficit-/hyperactivity disorder) is a mental disorder that affects a person's ability to pay attention a control impulse behavior. It has two parts; inattention and hyperactivity or impulsivity. The inattention is when a person is having a problem staying focus, forgetful of task, unable to handle small details and seems to not listen. The hyperactivity is frigidity or constant moving, not being able to sit still or for periods of time, talkative, fighting, making careless mistakes, failure to follow instructions, failure to fish what is started, organizational problems, becoming distracted, daydreaming, loss of time and speaking out often interrupting others. These symptoms vary according to the individual. It is not unusual for everyone to experience symptoms of forgetfulness, being bored but ADHD look to the frequency, intensity and interfere with normal activity. ADHD is not just a childhood diagnosis but can also relate to adults. In adults it is shown by poor organization, not completing task, thrill seeking, bad decision-making, inability to complete forms, returning call, keeping appointments and inability to concentrate. These could also be signs of depression, anxiety and other learning disabilities. If any of these symptoms exist seek professional help. Some people live a lifetime with undiagnosed and untreated ADHD. Ohers may find themselves with other mental disorders from the stress of undiagnosed ADHD, career lost or failures and bad relationships with other people. Both genetic and environmental factors have a bearing on a diagnosis of ADHD. There are no known cures for ADHD. It can be controlled with a combination of medicine and psych-therapist. Do not rely on non-professional diagnosis but seek professional help.

The mental health professional is known as a Clinical Mental Health Counselor, Psychologist, Psychiatrist, and Social Worker who are called psycho-therapist and conduct psycho-therapy the minimum qualification is a Master's Degree with continual annual training, adherence to a code of ethics and in some states a licensing board.

The people involved in diagnosing and helping you child can be a teacher, parent, physician and psych-therapist. No one want to label a child with a psychiatric disorder. In the past psychiatric disorders have been shameful and the person was ridiculed, scolded, and seen as hopeless. NOT THE CASE NOW!!!

If your child is in daycare, pre-school, or higher learning stop and take the time to talk to the teacher. Be pro-active. The teacher sees your child action a large part of the day as they do the academics, social interactions and life skill building traits. Learn to ask questions. Tell the teacher your concerns and ask for help in their observations of your child. Children can be diagnosed as young as four years of age. Most children are active and energetic at this age and a determination is very difficult to make. If you suspect ADHD, seek a professional help. In these years of growth, it is possible to misdiagnose ADHD for other problems like disciplinary, quietness and good behavior.

Stop and talk with the child's pediatrician. Be honest about what is seen in your child behavior. Give the pediatrician permission to share information with the therapist and vice/versa. Use recommended therapist and pediatricians.

Parent be honest. Stop and talk to yourself, spouse, significant other or grandparents about the child conduct and can give an accurate history of family behavior. This is history is important and could help in a diagnosis. Seek information about ADHD and guidance from a professional. Openly admit any short coming or need to improve parenting skills. No one was born a perfect parent but parenting skills can be learned.

The most important person in the treatment of a child with ADHD is the parent or caregiver. The parent could observe, teach, enforce and report the child activity. A child with a positive diagnosis of ADHD makes this task a very difficult job in that it is stressful, requiring additional time with the child, special attention to the child and specially making other children and family members aware of the condition.

Page purposefully left blank for your notes and plans. Use it!!!!!!!

FEAR

There is nothing to fear with ADHD. You can handle it and be successful at handling the illness, ADHD. Say it until you have adjusted to the sound of your voice acknowledging that your child has ADHD. Scream it, challenge it and conqueror it. It is important that you believe in yourself, your child therapist and your medication. Your child is depending on you. This is not a stranger, a disease or someone who is an alien, but your child. This is your son or daughter diagnosed with a treatable illness who need your love and attention. There are many famous people who suffered with ADHD. Many professionals that you deal with in your everyday life that have been diagnosed with ADHD. They have worked hard to control it. ADHD can be controlled and you can do it. Do not fear ADHD but challenge ADHD and overcome it. You are in control! The illness does not dictate your child's life.

Acceptance is the first element of control. Yes, accept it, wear it and handle it. The acceptance of a child with a mental disorder especially ADHD is necessary for complete treatment. They are different but need additional help with simple things. These children need additional hugs, kisses, attention and time. Issues involving children with psychological disorders are seldom resolved with only medication and psychological therapy. They need love and care. Many times, issues are masked by the medication. Therapist have limited time with your child. Teachers are overwhelmed with the classroom work. The primary difference is made by you as a parent. Tell your employer, "my child has ADHD and I may need to leave work early on some days or come in late some morning". Talk with your spouse and say, "we may need to give our child additional time, hugs and compliment for their accomplishments." Become proactive and include those around you. This is your child, DONOT BE AFRAID TO ASK FOR HELP FROM WHOEVER. Get the support of everyone and exclude no one.

Psycho-therapy and medication are not permanent healer. Healing requires a combination of medicine, psychotherapy and parental involvement. It is alright to for parents to fear psychotherapy and medicine, initially. It is not alright not to learn their benefits and make them available to your child. The fear is because of a lack of understanding and a time of grief for their child. Get the knowledge necessary to help your child. Know the medication and side effects. Do not put the child on a medication that you cannot pronounce and do not know the side effect or why this medication is prescribed by the doctor as the best treatment. Talk with the psycho-therapist and ask questions. Write down the questions and inquire. Ask for alternative treatment resources, updates to treatment process and volunteer to help. Ask to sit in the session periodically with the child. This is your child. Knowledge is critical to their success.

This is a treatable illness. Recognize and Embrace it. Analyze ADHD and love the desire to change it This is not a death sentence but a diagnosis that need understanding, acceptance and support. My child requires my undivided attention not only because of the ADHD but because this is my child. Teach yourself and teach your child My child requires my understanding to change their behavior. Be available, associate other parents who can provide a support network. It is a challenge but it is also your child well-being. Publicize and celebrate their successes and plan and work on their failures.

ADHD

Attention-Deficit-Hyperactive Disorder

ADHD is much like any other illness. Early detection is early treatment. If you have the slightest feeling something is wrong—it usually is so get help. ADHD is a mental illness that affect a person paying attention. It is impulsive behavior, lack of focus, forgetfulness, not listening, frigidity, talkative, squirming and loud talking. It is not just bad behavior, disrespectful behavior that makes you as a parent angry, and fed up. It is an illness that you with professional help can correct. At this writing there is no none cue but treatment may help reduce symptoms and improve life functioning skills.

A child's culture plays a part in ADHD diagnosis. Every child is not the same. Every household is not the same. Every parent is not the same. DO NOT compare your child or household to anyone else. You are who you are. Success is not defined by what happened in someone else's home, although the sharing of information can be beneficiary. Talk to other parents and share information both successes and failures. DO NOT COMPARE CHILDREN!!! It is important that you seek out a therapist who will take the time to listen, be empathetic, non-judgmental and tell you the truth. Do not be afraid to talk and confide in the therapist. Write down your questions before the session. If the therapist does not know the answer immediately, ask if they would research the issue for you. There may be a cost, PAY IT. The information is worth it. This is your child.

Parents should look for signs of behavior problems. Early signs, late signs are not to be ignored. Parents get a professional diagnosis and leave those attempted to be done by none-professionals persons where they are made. Get clear understanding of what is normal childhood behavior. If you have any doubt or need an opinion seek a professional advice. Different children behave differently so acknowledge these differences in watching children behavior. In fact, most children reflect their own parent behavior. If you were not a saint, it is possible but unlikely you will produce one. Children are not perfect; you were not. They are curious, noisy, active, full of energy, playful, prone to lie, cheat, steal and about a thousand other things. Look for the extremes, out of the ordinary conduct. Children with ADHD struggle to be like other children and they can be, with your help. They are frigidity, easily angered, and sometimes seems so troublesome but these are signs and symptoms that can be changed if they are not ignored.

The key to successful control of ADHD is knowledge. Know the illness and learn the remedies and utilize what you learn. You cannot fail, but there are times you grow weary. Take a break, refresh yourself and go back to solving the issue at hand.

Remember parents, it is alright to confront your child. Confrontation is the beginning of healing. Bad behavior is not cute, laughable and should be re-enacted or encouraged. It should be stopped immediately. Confrontation should not be harsh, demeaning or destructive but stern enough that the child knows the behavior is not acceptable. ADHD is not an excuse for bad behavior. This is your child and your desire is what is best for your child. Convey this message to the child at every opportunity. Remember your child know your triggers and hot button. They have make a reasonable study of you. It sounds laughable, but the child knows how to get attention from you. Be honest with your child and tell them how you feel about their behavior. There is no penalty for lack of knowledge. Say I do not know if you do not know but do not lie because they know. Mutual respect is very important in helping the child overcome obstacles paced in their lives by ADHD

TREATMENT FOR ADHD

Treatment for ADHD include medication, therapy, education, and most times a combination of all three. Medication may include: stimulants which increase the brain chemical dopamine which helps with the thinking and attention processes; non-stimulants which may improve focus, attention and impulsivity. Non-stimulant is slow to work and do not have as many side effects as stimulants. Therapy is provided by a mental health professional can help with ADHD with developing skills, providing appropriate training and education, stress management, support groups, and better coping with everyday issues. There is no one treatment for ADHD. Treatment is sought to reduce symptoms and develop coping skills.

Psycho-therapy for parent and child

Psycho-therapy simply means "I need to talk with someone about what is bothering me" "I need to focus" improve my livelihood, well-being and mental disorder. Most therapy that works for the child will also work for the parents. This is the beginning of a relationship between parent and child to, learn together, work together and become successful together. Psycho-therapy helps the individual identify strengths, identify weaknesses and provide education. The child and parent together learn coping skills and ways to reduce ADHD symptoms. Psycho-therapy alone or coupled with medication is not a cure but a help with managing the ADHD. One of the simplest therapy for ADHD children is STC (stop-think-choose)

A child with ADHD body and mind is active, constantly moving, full of energy and unstoppable. Stopping anything becomes a learned behavior. Gently hold the child by the hand and look eyeball to eyeball with a kindness and say, "I need you to stop for a moment"

This works for the parent also in observing and reacting to the child's behavior. When ADHD behavior is seen the parent should stop before reacting'

Think about your response before responding to the child. No, not always, you are human and do not forget that. Every word should be but is not always pleasant. In this case parents

make a choice that is beneficial to you, not the child. Think about what you are going to say and how to best say it. Try to listen to yourself while speaking but do not speak in fear. If the statement comes out harsh do not be afraid to apologize. It is a learning process for the child and parent.

MAKING CHOICES

All children need to learn how to make choices. Children diagnosed with ADHD must learn to make choices. It is not automatic, choice (decision-making) is a learned skill. Choice requires knowledge. Choice is important because it benefits parent and child with thinking, calculation and decision-making. Parents, teachers and care-givers **must** understand that children diagnosed with ADHD cannot always make even simple decision. Helping with decision-making is very important in handling children with ADHD. Once a good decision is made the choice will help their self-esteem, A bad decision can help with the thought process in helping them walk thru the decision and make a negative a positive.

Choice has consequences:

Make consequences reasonable--These are children with ADHD. In helping them to make decisions there must be consequences and rewards both for good and bad behavior. It should always be kept in mind that you are the parent. Take control and be patience. The child will challenge your authority. Do not withhold or delay the reward There should be a balance. Parents learn to reward yourself and if here are other children in the family allow them to share in the reward system. It builds family unity.

Make sure that parent and child understand the consequences and rewards in helping children with ADHD it is important to know the benefits of following the rules and consequences for failure from the beginning. Consequences and rules should not be made as you go along or changed without explanation and agreement of both parent and child. Everyone should understand at the onset what the consequences and rules are.

Enforce the consequences—Do not change the consequences bad or good. Parents leave your feelings and heart out of it. It is hard to do but try anyway. Explain why or why not' challenge the child and parent accept the challenge from your child.

Basic Rules for handling ADHD:

> Rules are what helps control behavior. Rules will not be effective unless they are understood, agreed to and enforced. With ADHD children, there must be standard rules for behavior and expectations. All parties should know the rules. Hearing the rules are not the same as knowing and agreeing to the rules. Everyone should hear and acknowledge an understanding of the rules. Sign a document, recite the rule and tell the other person what your understanding about that rule and repeat the process until everyone understand.

There must be a meeting of the minds on rules for everyone. All persons must agree to what constitute a violation of the rules and the consequences for any violations. It is important to practice active listening and clearly define expectations and goals to the child. If there is a reward do what you say when the goal has been reached.

Parents should structure task to fit the child and provide positive talk whether task is completed or not. Concentrate on the effort not the completion sometimes. The smaller the task, the greater the number of successful completions. Task should be increased according to the child's ability not parent's expectations.

Enforce the rules. Methods of enforcement of the rules should be pre-determined. Many times parent will be overwhelmed by the efforts of child or the whims of a child and change the rules. Don't do it! Take your emotions out of enforcement. Children are good at manipulating their parents. Parents have a soft heart toward their children.

Do not allow your child to use the fact of being diagnosed with ADHD as an excuse for bad behavior. Expect the best always, in fact demand it.

Explain why the child should work harder to maintain good grades and a positive attitude.

Do not reward everything but reward and acknowledge the child overcoming challenges

Do not separate the children in the household but seek common behavior and encourage unity.

Parents take a break! it is alright to acknowledge that you cannot handle it that day.

Medication for ADHD

There are many medications to treat ADHD. Medication is not a cure all, but it reduced and help symptoms. Medication helps increase the child's alertness and attention. The medication sometimes improves communication of parts of the brain by a process called neurotransmission. Many ADHD medications are addictive and work for only a short period of time. Doctors, therapist and researchers have stated "there is no known cure." It does not mean they have given up on finding one, just that honesty is the best policy. Now that we know that let's work on reduction of the negative behavior. Everyone that encounters your child becomes a helper.

REMEMBER TO ONLY GIVE YOUR CHILD MEDICATION THAT IS PRESCRIBED FOR THEM: DONOT SHARE MEDICATION: DONOT INCREASE OR DECREASE THE DOSAGE WITHOUT THE DOCTOR PERMISSION!!!!!

Many of the medications are addictive and has side effects. Understand the side effects and reasons for the medication. Talk to the therapist and doctors until you have good information. Explain the side effects of the medication to your child often. Parents monitor the child for evidence of side effects. Parent help the child to recognize the side effects and help the child to overcome them. Do not allow the use the side effect as an excuse for bad conduct, but use them to overcome bad conduct.

This booklet cannot explore all the different medication for the treatment of ADHD. Researchers are constantly evaluating different medications, and finding new ones. When it becomes necessary to place your child on medication do not rebel, but excel. Ask questions, read literature, and be mindful of the child's response to medication. This is your child and you have a right to know why this medication, what this medication does and the good/bad effects of any medication. There should be no surprises and if there are YOU report them to the doctor or therapist immediately. If your doctor or therapist is non-responsive, confront them respectfully and ask why? Do not be afraid to change therapist or doctors, ask for a second opinion or ask to be a part of the therapy session.

Many side effects, decreased appetite sleeping disorder mild anxiety and restlessness.

Medications used to treat AHD are stimulants which increase brain chemical dopamine and helps thinking and attention; non-stimulants which improve focus, attention and impulsivity; antidepressants are usually with adults. only use medications that are prescribed by a doctor and only give the prescribed dosages.

TEACHER/DOCTOR/THERAPIST

The teacher is one of the most important person in your child life. In many cases teachers are the first to recognize the symptoms of ADHD, they do not diagnose but can tell you what they see. Accept their observations and see a professional. This booklet cannot express the value of teachers and their help in dealing with a diagnosis of ADHD. You have one child to contend with and think of the frustration you have, while a teacher may have four or five in a classroom setting for eight hours a day five day a week. The teacher need to know all children diagnosed with ADHD. The help and understanding a teacher gives your child has a lot to do with cooperation and information from the parent. Teacher need to know if your child has or you suspect your child of having ADHD. They need to know the medication, amount taken and durations. Tell them who your child therapist is and what intervention is being used for changed behavior. It is important that open dialogue between the teacher and parent be maintained. This allows the teacher to focus on your child positive behavior, change expectations as needed and give you correct information.

Ten things that might help a teacher with ADHD children:

1. Always avoid singling out the child with ADHD and look for positive strengths:
2. Ge help to learn behavior modification methods
3. Let the children dump their backpacks
4. Post classroom rules and enforce them
5. As for feedback from students
6. Do daily physical activities
7. Set up a token and reward system
8. Look at 504 and IEP plans stop the open giving of medication.

Children with ADHD are always stand out in the classroom setting. They demand attention, speak out of order, have problems with following instructions, easily forget, do not complete homework, have bad motor skills and have a problem with organization.

Doctor

The child's pediatrician should be consulted for all medical decisions including behavior. If you feel that your child is exhibiting extreme behavior call the pediatrician. Do not substitute your judgment for that of a professional. It is important to give the pediatrician correct information. Parents, write down in detail your concerns before the appointment, be prepared to give examples of bad behavior, take time to understand the diagnosis and treatment prescribed including medication and finally check back in thirty days and inform the heath care person of the effects of medication or treatment.

Therapist

A good therapist is important to the successful treatment of your child. The therapist should have proper credentials and training. The therapist will do an evaluation and diagnoses of your child based on sound medical evidence. Most therapist will do a detail intake interview and testing prior to any treatment. Therapist with a child may also include treatment for the parent. The therapist will explain an intervention and treatment plan for your child.

The goal of therapy is to enforce the positive and manage or eliminate the negative behavior. Therapy should teach management skills and strategies. In most cases therapy is as effective as medication. A therapist because of the length of time for treatment is more methodical, mentally invasive of the person.

Parents should look for certain qualities in the therapist. A therapist and the parent should be able to establish a therapeutic relationship of empathy. genuineness and trust. The therapist should be motivated, goal oriented, able to express themselves, and explain the symptoms of different intervention and mental illness. The therapist should be cultural sensitive, flexible and able to instill hope and optimism. In most instances your doctor or school officials can recommend a capable therapist. Parent do not be afraid to talk to the therapist. If you do not develop a good therapeutic relationship, it is alright to change therapist. This is not a one therapist fit all situation.

Things Not to Say to An ADHD CHILD

Part of therapy is to promote good self-esteem and a positive image for a person with ADHD. The best parent often says things hurtful or in anger. Once words are out, it is difficult to change them or their meaning. Children with ADHD are very sensitive and the most loving parents if not careful can say things that are later regretted.

Example:

Do not say these phrases….

"_____ is very bright but he never finish anything" "I stand over _____ until he complete all assignment……… you irritate me…..dummy……you are stupid…………….you are not normal….you are just like your father or mother……..you are lazy….you want a check…..you can do betters……… you just need a whopping……That's stupid   you are a trouble-maker

I do not want to hear from you again unless I call on you………that crazy…. you are good for nothing……. you don't act like other kids……Don't try to be a show-off   you goofball, you loser, can you stop fidgeting   are you ever on time

Words hurt and the effect linger for a lifetime. It is important that we are careful about what we say, the tone in which it is said and time. TAKE A BREAK!!!!! When handling ADHD children it is important to do self-care. TAKE A MOMENT FOR SELF!!!!!

CONCLUSION

You are not alone. Every parent knows the angry, defiant and disruptive behavior of those diagnosed with ADHD. Treatment starts with learning control. Parent do not take the diagnosis personally. Try to stay calm, work with the therapist and be consistent. There is no single test—no single treatment- no single therapy for your child. The successful treatment for any childhood disorder are proper diagnosis, medication if necessary, early detection, knowledge, patience and love. The patience to wait on the treatment process to work and the endless love for your child despite the diagnosis. Children with ADHD need love but so do your other children so make love, kindness and forgiveness an across the board family quality. It is the best treatment.

It is never too early to look for ADHD. If suspected, set an appointment with a professional, be honest about your suspicion and accept the diagnosis. Parents should look for what is called signs such as inattention, hyperactivity and impulsivity. The symptoms must be present for six months couple with non-age appropriate activities. Do not self-diagnose. Make an appointment with psychiatrist, psychologist, clinical mental health counselor and pediatrician.

Parents do not mistake bad behavior for ADHD and do not excuse bad behavior because of ADHD. There is no none cure but there is control and reduction of the symptoms. ADHD has no economic, social, political or cultural boundaries. ADHD is not gender or age specific. It is a mental diagnosis that can be controlled in most cases by therapy and medication.

Resources:

www.help4adhd.org   1800-233-4050   www.cdc.gov/ncbddd/adhd/

www.nimh.nih.gov/findhelp   www.mentalhealth.gov

clinicaltrials.gov   www.understand.org

www.edgefoundation.org

https://www.nim.nih.gov/medlineplus/attentiondeficithyperactivitydisorder.htm

http://idea.ed.gov/.   www.adhdadulthood.com

Contact your local mental health authority.

WORKING TOGETHER AND USING ALL AVALIABLE RESOURCES FOR OUR CHILDREN DIAGNOSED WITH

ADHD

WE ARE WINNING!!!!!!!!!!

AND THAT IS ALL THAT MATTERS

This book is dedicated to all the parents, teachers, therapist, pediatricians, psychologist, psychiatrist and staff workers who make a difference in the life of our children with or without a diagnosis of ADHD. The children are successful because of YOU!!!!

www.ingramcontent.com/pod-product-compliance
Lightning Source LLC
Chambersburg PA
CBHW050039230526
45470CB00003B/1338